Table of Contents

Introduction

Before you get started, you need to understand the difference between cannabis oil and CBD oil. One has THC, and one does not. This means that cannabis oil, which contains THC, can produce a high. However, CBD oil does not have THC, and it does not produce a high. Of course, there is more than just the two. You'll learn all about what makes up cannabis, what uses both CBD oil and cannabis oil have, the variations they come from, and much more. The goal of this book is so that you can make the right choices to help with your own medical conditions or use CBD oil to help with general, preventative measures to keep your body healthy.

The Varieties

Cannabinoids describe the various compounds found in cannabis, also known as marijuana. You have THC, CBD, CBG, and CBC. As mentioned in the introduction, THC gets you high. Cannabinoids doesn't have a role in the plant's development. However, they metabolites act as the immune system or the plants.

THC

This binds to the cannabinoid receptors present in your brain, which allows it to work with your central nervous system. This produces psychoactive effects. Not everyone responds to THC in the same way. Some people are calm and peaceful. Other people get anxious and paranoid. It all depends on the chemistry of your body and what strain or even the concentration of the THC you've consumed. You can have a negative experience with a particular strain or even a high concentration, but you may still want to try a different strain or even a lower concentration.

If you're going to be using THC, it's better to start with a low concentration and take it slow. Cannabis lasts for several hours, but it can also take several hours to take effect depending on the strain you're using. If you don't feel anything after a half hour, you'll still want to wait. Do not immediately get more and assume it isn't working. Various strains can cause the following in different people.

- Paranoia
- Red Eyes
- Relaxation
- Sedation
- Pain Relief
- Memory Impairment
- Laughter
- Anxiety
- Increased heart rate
- Feeling heavy
- Hunger
- Elation

- Dry mouth
- Energy
- Dizziness
- Drowsiness

Long term effects have not been documented or researched well, and the side effects are heavily debated. Some people believe that long term exposure to THC can lead to an increased tolerance. Bronchitis can be a long term side effect if THC is consumed through the inhalation of smoke. This is why THC infused products have become popular, including the vapor form.

THC is known to benefit the following conditions as well.

- Crohn's Disease
- ADHD
- Arthritis
- Cancer
- Chronic Pain
- Appetite Loss
- ADHD
- Alzheimer's
- Glaucoma
- Inflammation
- Insomnia
- Multiple Sclerosis (MS)
- Sleep Apnea
- PTSD
- Neuropathic Pain
- Nausea
- Migraines
- Fibromyalgia

The most common way to consume THC is through smoking marijuana. However, there are also edible THC products. Edibles can be just as intoxicating as smoking it, and some people find that they're more affected by using edibles rather than smoking.

CBD

There are many medicinal benefits that CBD has that overlap with THC, so you can get the benefits without the high. This includes pain, inflammation, and anxiety. CBD is not intoxicating, and it can be sold over the counter, allowing you to purchase it without a Medical Marijuana card in most states. Remember that since it cannot get you high, CBD products do not have the same regulations as THC products. They're often referred to as hemp products instead of cannabis products or even marijuana products.

Even in states that do not allow for either the medical or recreational use of marijuana, most of them will allow for the purchase of CBD products. However, that doesn't make them easy to find. If medical or recreational marijuana is legal in your state, then CBD oil is guaranteed to be legal as well, but that doesn't mean they're sold at the local pharmacy. You will have to find a place to purchase them, and many people turn online for just that.

CBD oil can be extracted from both hemp plants and marijuana plants, but if it's extracted from a marijuana plant it'll have a trace amount of THC. The exact level will decide if it's legal or not. The THC level usually has to be under one percent, but there are some states that require it to be less than 0.3 percent. However, places like Delaware allow up to five percent in CBD products while still allowing them to be legal. Five percent is not enough to cause intoxication.

Research has shown that CBD that's extracted from marijuana plants instead of hemp plants is more effective. This is because it has other cannabinoids that it can work with to make it more effective. The strongest and commonly recommended strains of CBD are ACDC, Remedy, Harlequin, Katelyn Faith, Cannatonic, and Charlotte's Web. They contain a high level of CBD, but some do contain a high level of THC as well, so be careful which strain you purchase depending on where you are. These are the best strains due to their medicinal benefits, but they may not be available over the counter where you live.

To understand how it works, you need to understand that your body has a network of neurons that is referred to as the endocannabinoid system. This has various receptions that bind the cannabinoids you ingest, such as CBD, but we don't know much about the interactions between the receptors. This system is connected to other major systems in our bodies. Which is why cannabis as well as marijuana have various medicinal benefits.

Some studies support that CBD is effect in treating epilepsy as well as their seizure disorders. Other studies have shown that CBD can treat various neurological diseases such as Alzheimer's, Parkinson's, and Multiple Sclerosis as well. CBD can also help to protect your nerve cells, which is referred to as a neuroprotective effect. This is why it's such a great tool in fighting neurodegenerative disorders. Though, the most common use for CBD is chronic pain. It's become a popular alternative to prescription painkillers, including opioids.

The pain relieving effects of CBD can be compared to morphine, and it has been in many studies. It has even been found to work well with morphine, allowing your doctor to prescribe you smaller doses of morphine, as it also reduces the effects of the drug. Some studies have shown CBD oil also inhibits tumor growth, which allows it to slow cancer growth, including lung, prostate, colon, and breast cancer. Since cancer cells rely on rapid regeneration, CBD can also effectively kill off cancer cells in some people. Since the cells cannot overwhelm the immune system, then your immune system is able to fight off the cancer cells more effectively.

Both CBD and THC have anti-inflammatory properties as well. CBD and THC have been known to help with emotional and mood disorders as well. CBD can help you to increase your ability to forget a traumatic memory or event, especially those that cause PTSD. It does not completely erase the memory of the event, but it makes it easier for you to let go of the memory and stop focusing on it. It can also help with depression, agoraphobia, anxiety and other mental or emotional conditions. CBD can also calm the mind and assist in the production of serotonin, which is considered a happy chemical of the brain.

CBD will not get you high, as we previously discussed, but you can use CBD along with THC. CBD helps to counterbalance the intoxication of THC. So if you are experiencing too much intoxication, anxiety or paranoid, you can increase your amount of CBD that you ingest along with THC. This helps to soften the overall experience, making it more pleasant for people who are sensitive to the effects of THC, since THC affects everyone differently.

You can find CBD oil, which is a popular way to purchase CBD, but you can also purchase beauty products, and topical ointments. CBD oil is recommended to be used, which can be used in a vaporizer. You'll find it's usually compressed into a wax form, and then it's placed in a small cartridge and warmed by the vaporizer's battery. This creates a vapor that you then inhale, which is much like nicotine vaporizers.

However, if you do not want to use CBD oil, the next recommended product to get the medicinal effects you're looking for is to find it in an edible product such as food, beverages or tinctures. Tinctures are a flavored oil, which can be applied to the tongue or under the tongue by a dropper. Edibles are extremely popular since you can get them from drinks, to cookies to candy bars. They're easy to consume, and many people find it hard to taste the CBD in it.

CBD oils are also used in pet products, including dog treats to help with anxiety, joint pain and more. CBD powders can be found too, which are usually flavored and can be sprinkled into your dog's food. However, make sure that you do your research. There are many companies out there that will simply imply that the product has THC or CBD, but they don't actually contain any of either.

CBC & CBG

CBC is also called cannabichromene, and very little is known about it. Fifty years ago CBC was discovered, and it branches off from CBG. CBC is also not intoxicating, just like CBD, and it does not bind well to the CB1 receptor. This is why you'll find a euphoric high when it's ingested, but it doesn't bind well to two pain receptors either TRPA1 or TRPV1. CBC works best when it's not used on its own. It should be paired with other cannabinoids such as THC or CBD. It does work independently, but it's not nearly as effective. Studies are limited on CBC, but some studies show that it has an acute effect on slowing down the growth and development of new cancer cells.

However, CBG is even more effective. CBC has also been known to relieve chronic inflammation and pain, but not nearly as well as CBD. CBC also has a powerful effect on depression, especially when paired with THC. CBC can also be found in some creams, since it's known to reduce various types of acne. CBG is found in small quantities, and it's not intoxicating. CBG isn't present in high quantities given current strains of marijuana, but cannabis breeders are now trying to produce strains with higher quantities of CBG.

CBG is most effective in treating intraocular pressure or glaucoma. CBG can also reduce the inflammation associated with inflammatory bowel disease. It can also help to prevent nerve cell degeneration, which mean it's a neuroprotection. It can also help to fight against tumors, just like CBC, CBD and THC.

CBN

CBN, also known as Cannabinol, comes out once the dried plant flower starts to become stale. If you leave it sitting, the CBN will multiply in it. CBN stimulates your appetite, and it has pain-relieving benefits, just like THC. CBN relaxes blood vessels and helps to release endorphins. CBN can also treat asthma because it has anti-inflammatory effects. It can also help to boost your immune system, which can help with asthma related to allergies too. CBN also has sedative properties, and it's considered to be as effective as Valium. Those suffering from glaucoma can also benefit from CBN since it helps to lower ocular pressure, which is what causes blindness.

Hemp Oil vs. CBD Oil

While CBD oil may be called hemp oil, it doesn't mean that all hemp oil is CBD oil. You'll need to research the product carefully if you want to use a CBD oil labeled hemp oil. In this chapter, we'll go over the differences and what to look for.

True Hemp Oil

Hemp oil comes from a plant known as hemp, so the extract is taken from the seeds. The type of oil extracted from all plants in the cannabis genus can produce this type of oil. However, industrial hemp is the only plant that's used for real hemp oil. The amount of psychoactive substances in it are contained at a minimal level that will not affect most people. It's great for cooking, and it'll provide you with various nutrients. It provides a nutty and crisp flavor, and it's a great replacement for olive oil for salads and certain recipes. It can also be a great natural moisturizer, which many people use after showering. It can also be used as a base for plastic, used in the production of paints, and it can even be used as bio-diesel. Hemp oil is also used in the making of some soaps and lotions.

True CBD Oil

You already know that CBD oil is a short term for cannabidiol oil. It's a natural component of both hemp and cannabis. It's made from the stalks, leaves, and flowers of hemp, but it is not made from the seeds like hemp oil. The benefits and uses of CBD oil has already been discussed.

The Difference

The difference between marijuana and hemp is the THC content. Hemp oil contains a low level of CBD, which is less than twenty-five parts per million, and CBD oil can be up to fifteen percent CBD. There are some people marketing hemp oil as a medicinal product, but the medicinal benefits of hemp oil is negligible. Here are a few of the key differences.

The natural source of the product is the most notable difference. The seeds from hemp are cold pressed to extract oil to make hemp oil. CBD oil is produced from the cannabis sativa plant, and as stated before it's produced from the leaves, flowers and stalks. High-tech extraction or solvents are used to draw the CBD from the plant. This is why the chemical makeup of both oils is notably different.

CBD oil has a similar chemical makeup to THC containing marijuana, which is why it's able to help with so many medical conditions. However, hemp seed oil only contains fatty acids, minerals and vitamins, which can be found in most healthy oils. This doesn't mean that one is better than the other, but that each has unique properties and uses. So, overall you'll find that while hemp oil is healthy it won't affect you in any other way. However, CBD oil affects your endocannabinoid system, which helps a variety of conditions.

CBD Oil FAQ

Before we learn more about CBD oil, let's first take a look at some frequently asked questions and their answers.

Is it legal everywhere in the US?

It depends on the type of CBD oil that you buy. Just make sure that it has no THC or less THC than your state's cap, and then it's legal. Most CBD oil is legal because the THC is under one percent, so just look into the product before you buy it. Even five percent of THC is not enough to get you high, but it may be enough to make that particular brand of CBD oil illegal in your area. If this is the case, then just look for a different CBD oil.

Do I need a prescription for CBD oil?

No, you don't need a prescription to get CBD oil. You do want to discuss with your doctor that you're taking CBD oil to make sure that it doesn't negatively impact any other medications you're taking or health conditions you may have.

How long do I have to wait for it to take effect?

How long it takes for CBD oil to take effect will depend on your particular extract as well as the dosage. It should only take twenty to thirty minutes to see noticeable effects with most problems, including chronic pain. However, remember that CBD oil can also be taken in food as a preventive, and in this case you'd be looking for long term effects and not short term effects.

Do you experience any form of high from CBD oil?

No CBD oil should contain enough THC for you to get a high from it. If you're making your own CBD oil and you experience a high, then you did not extract your CBD from the cannabis properly.

Can I just juice raw cannabis to get CBD oil?

No, CBD oil will not come from juicing raw cannabis. However, you will have CBD come out, but you'll also have high levels of THC come out, which means that you aren't just getting the CBD that CBD oil provides.

Is one CBD product better than the other?

While you can have one brand of CBD oil that's better than another because it has a higher concentration or purity, one product is not better than the next. It all depends on what you're using it for. For example, if you're going to use it for eczema, you're going to want to have a CBD product such as a slave. Though, if you're looking to use it as a preventive method, you may want to bake with it. This means you just need CBD oil. Just figure out what product is best for your specific needs, but normal CBD oil is the most versatile.

About Rick Simpson Oil

If you've been reading about medical marijuana, you've likely heard the term Rick Simpson oil. This is also often referred to as RSO, which is a highly concentrate cannabis oil, which does have medical benefits. This type of cannabis oil is also able to benefit people suffering from cancer, so let's look at the story behind it.

Where It Came From

Rick Simpson was an engineer in Canada in the year 1997. He worked in the boiler room of a hospital, and it had toxic fumes and poor ventilation, which was a bad combination that wrecked his nervous system. This gave him a temporary shock which caused him to fall off a ladder and hit his head on the way down. When he came to, he contacted co-workers to help him get to the ER, but he suffered ear ringing and dizziness for some time after the accident occurred.

The medication prescribed to him had little to no affect, and his own symptoms seemed to worsen. After watching a documentary on medical cannabis, which caused him to ask his doctor about medical marijuana. The doctor didn't want to consider medical marijuana as an option, so Rick Simpson decided to research the matter on his own. When he started to use it, it decreased his tinnitus significantly as well as improving some of his other symptoms.

His Cancer Diagnosis

Years later after the new millennium, he noticed three bumps located on his arm, and the doctor thought they may be cancerous. After having them tested, they discovered it was indeed skin cancer. Rick Simpson had experienced success with his previous use of cannabis for his condition, and he had already heard that THC could kill off cancer cells in lab mice. This led him to use it again, so he treated the bumps on his arm topically.

He placed the cannabis oil onto a bandage, leaving it there for a few days. After four days, he removed the bandages, and he noticed that the growths were already gone. His doctor still refused to admit that cannabis was a better treatment than the conventional methods. However, Rick Simpson believed in the miracle that was his cannabis oil, so he started to cultivate his own strain. He harvested it, creating a unique concentration, where is where Rick Simpson Oil came from.

The Persecution

Rick then wanted to distribute the oil to people in need, and he didn't want to charge. He helped to treat over 5,000 people with his oil, but it had its struggles and setbacks. Rick Simpson was persecuted in Canada, and his house was raided by law authorities multiple times. Due to the raids he lost thousands of plants, but he wanted to stick to his goal and continue helping people with cannabis oil. This is why Rick Simpson is considered a hero in the medical marijuana community.

Making Rick Simpson Oil

It isn't hard to make homemade Rick Simpson Oil, and it's similar to making cannabis butter or other infused oils. Indica is preferred for the best results, but you should base it on your unique condition. The following recipe will give you sixty grams to use, which is about a three month treatment regimen. If you're looking for a smaller treatment, then you can split up the recipe into smaller sections. A single ounce of cannabis will give you three to four grams for example.

Ingredients

- 1 lb. Cannabis (Quality Matters)
- 2 Gallons Solvent (such as 99 percent isopropyl alcohol)
- One 5 Gallon Bucket
- A Wooden Spoon
- A Cheesecloth
- 1 Deep Bowl
- A Rice Cooker
- 60 ml Catheter Tip Syringe, Plastic

Steps

Follow the instructions below, and make sure that you do them precisely.

1. Start by providing your dried cannabis into your bucket, pouring the solvent over it so that your cannabis is completely submerged.
2. Crush and stir your cannabis using your spoon as you add more solvent into your mix. You'll need to use a wooden spoon so that there isn't a reaction.
3. Continue to stir your mixture for a few minutes, so the THC gets dissolved into the liquid. About eight percent of this compound will be dissolved into the solvent liquid.
4. Use your cheesecloth to drain the liquid away from your cannabis, and then put your cannabis back into your bucket. Add more of the solvent liquid, and stir again for a few minutes, and then drain it from the plant matter using your cheesecloth again.

5. Throw away the cannabis, and then put your liquid into your rice cooker. Fill it up three-quarters full, and then turn it on. The rice cooker helps you to keep a slow and steady temperature. Your temperature can't get over 300 degrees F or you'll lose your cannabinoids by cooking off. This is why you shouldn't use a slow cooker or crockpot since it overheats the mixture easily. You also have to keep the temperature at a steady heat between 210 and 230 degrees F. this allows for decarboxylation, and your solvent liquid will evaporate steadily but slowly. Continue to add the mixture into the rice cooker, and make sure that you go at a gradual pace. You'll want to make sure that your rice cooker is kept in a well ventilated area, and it should be free of sparks, cigarettes, fire or stovetops. Remember that your solvent is combustible.

6. As soon as your solvent has completely evaporated, your oil can be put into a syringe, allowing you to use the correct dose easily. Your oil should be thick, which makes dispensing it hard. You'll want to place your syringe under hot water to help it flow easier.

Flavonoids & CBD Oil

Before you can understand the role that flavonoids play in CBD oil, you need to understand what flavonoids are. They are a nutrient family that has over 6,000 members. About twenty of the compounds in this family can be found in cannabis. They're known for their anti-inflammatory and antioxidant benefits, and they contribute to the color in many foods you eat. These flavonoids can be extracted from cannabis and then tested, and it's proven various therapeutic effects.

Flavonoids & CBD

Cannabis flavonoids play a large part in their flavor and odor for each marijuana strain varieties. The term flavonoids comes from the word flavus, which is Latin for yellow. It produces yellow, and red/blue in petals, which can attract pollinators. In cannabis, the flavonoids are called cannaflavins, which they provide taste, vibrant color, overall sensory experience and smell depending on the cannabis strain. The distribution of cannaflavins depends on the growing conditions and genetics of the plant.

People can now extract cannaflavins, allowing you to get a stronger sample, which also has a stronger smell and taste, which can be used to supplement normal cannabis consumption. They don't add to the high since cannaflavins are not psychoactive, but they do have relaxing effects similar to CBD. They also play an important role in the cultivation of cannabis, as they affect UV filtering and prevention of fungi and pests. Flavonoids are members of the nutrient family, as stated before, and they produce antioxidants in the cannabis. The plant has to be allowed to grow properly to get a full range of cannaflavins. They're currently being researched, but we do know a little about what they actually do.

An Overall Look

There is evidence to suggest that flavonoids work with CBD and THC to contribute to the effects that cannabis produces. This theory is called the entourage effect, which says that all compounds work together to affect the endocannabinoid system which allows for cannabis to affect your body. The flavonoids are though to subdue psychoactive properties in THC, and people are currently researching their therapeutic properties. Research suggests they're related to anti-inflammatory, anti-carcinogenic and anti-oxidative effects.

Cannaflavin A & B

These are found to be powerful anti-inflammatories. PGE-2 is commonly responsible for inflammation, which is exactly what cannaflavin A and B has been shown to inhibit, much like aspirin but much more powerful.

Catechins

You can also find catechins in cocoa, teas, pome fruits, as well as cannabis. It promotes a healthy cardiovascular system because it's anti-hypertensive, anti-oxidative, anti-proliferative and anti-inflammatory, which can help you to maintain a healthy cholesterol level.

Beta-Sitosterol

This is a cannabis flavonoid that's also found in avocados and nuts, and it has strong anti-inflammatory properties.

Quercetin

This can be found in many vegetables and fruits as well, and they're antiviral and contain antioxidants. The quercetin in cannabis has been known to inhibit the influenza A virus.

Vitexin & Isovitexin

These are shown to have anti-cancer effects. They're considered to be "chemo-preventive", and they help to encourage the degradation of cancerous cells.

Orientin

This is a flavonoid which is commonly extracted from plants, and it has various beneficial properties. It's anti-aging, anti-viral, and anti-bacterial, contains antioxidants, is anti-inflammatory, cardio-protective, radiation protective, contains vasodilation, neuroprotective, anti-depression, and anti-adipogenesis and has pain relieving properties.

An In Depth Look at Treatments

CBD oil and cannabis oil can treat a variety of conditions, but let's take a look at what just CBD oil can treat without having to go for straight cannabis oil. You can reap these benefits without the high THC causes!

Neck & Back Pain

One of the most common uses of both cannabis oil and CBD oil is for neck and back pain, which you'll find out more about in this chapter. Millions of people are plagued by neck and back pain around the world, and most treatments are simple at best, but they often don't work or at least don't heal the problem.

The worst part is that many medications that are prescribed for this type of pain can cause harm to other organs. Many people suffering from this type of pain seek out surgery in the hopes of relief when neuropathy and medications don't work. However, this can cause further complications or be too costly. When you go for a surgery you leave yourself open to various predicaments, but this isn't the case when you use CBD or cannabis oil.

You've probably seen a photo of a spine, and you'll known that they're made of discs formed with cartilage. This is meant to ensure that the bone isn't worn down from day to day activity. However, you can suffer decay from various factors including a lack of hydration, lack of oxygen, poor diet, or even chronic inflammation. Over one hundred million Americans suffer from neck and back pain, and most of them are treated using anti-inflammatory medicines, which are also known as NSAIDS. They're usually ibuprofen, valium, or muscle relaxers.

However even ibuprofen can lead to constipation and other gastro disorders including stomach ulcers. However, there has been a connection between cannabinoids and relief from neck and back pain. They can treat cartilage discs in the neck and back, which can lead to an overall decrease in pain. It can even result in regeneration of lost cells, which can help to improve your quality of everyday life, manage the chronic pain and promote healthy sleep.

Multiple Sclerosis

Also known as MS this disease will affect you for the rest of your life. It can affect everything from your spinal cord, brain, your optic nerves, and it can alter your balance. MS can also alter the way you see the world, how your body controls your muscles and your body's control of other bodily functions. Depending on the person, you may suffer different symptoms. Some people only have a few smaller symptoms that require little to no treatment, but others are struggling with MS to a degree that affects their daily lives.

Essentially, MS causes your immune system to attack myelin. Myelin is the fat substance that protects your nerve fibers. Your nerves become damaged without this myelin. This will lead to scar tissue, and some symptoms include struggling to walk, the inability to walk, fatigue, tingling in your feet and hands, sexual difficulties, blurred vision, muscle spasms, depression, overall pain and general weakness. Symptoms for MS usually show between twenty and thirty years.

These symptoms often get worse over time, but the cause of this condition is unknown. It's considered to be linked to genetics and smoking, but this isn't the only suspected causes. The treatment options for MS are also lacking. Therefore many people seek out CBD oil as a valid treatment option. It can help to reduce the amount of problems you have when trying to sleep, it can reduce daily pain, reduce daily spasms, and reduce the spastic muscle motions. Sadly, most of the knowledge we have of how CBD oil affects this condition is from various people's accounts.

Fibromyalgia

This is another condition involving chronic pain, and it can lead to musculoskeletal irritation which can cause a full-body pain. It can also cause cognitive disorders, and there is no current cure for this disease. Therefore, treatment is simply pain management, which is where CBD oil comes in handy. Currently fibromyalgia affects the lives of millions, and it affects the fibers in your body that feel pain they send the sensation back to your brain, forcing an overall sensation of pain and irritation.

You're more likely to suffer from fibromyalgia if you're a woman, and stress is considered a possible cause. Those that suffer with fibromyalgia are also more susceptible to other diseases including horrible migraines, irritable bowel syndrome and chronic fatigue. Luckily, the reason CBD oil works for this condition is because fibromyalgia actually uses the endocannabinoid system, which is the same system that CBD oil does.

CBD oil interferes with this system, which decreases the amount of pain you feel from fibromyalgia. It does this by binding the microglial cells and reducing the number of cytokines in your bloodstream. When someone usually treats fibromyalgia they either suffer other problems which causes you to take more medicine, such as with migraines, which will cause more side effects. For wore cases opioid pain medications as well as corticosteroids are used, which has its own problems, including the possibility of addiction.

CBD oil helps to offer you treatment without the side effects of the various other treatments or medicines that could do you more harm than good. However, just because some patients find relief in CBD oil to treat fibromyalgia, you should keep in mind that it won't last forever. However, since there are little to no side effects of CBD oil, it's a valid choice to try.

Keep in mind that there isn't much known about fibromyalgia, so each case is different and needs to be treated accordingly. Some research has suggested that many cases of fibromyalgia is due to a deficient endocannabinoid system, where it's unable to regulate the appetite, pain, sleep, mood, sexual patterns and inflammation of your body. Since CBD oil directly affects this system, it can help to set your system back to normal patterns. Below you'll find some of the best types of CBD oil used to treat fibromyalgia.

- **CBD Pure:** All pure extracts have different levels of potency. They continuously work on their formula so that they can achieve a higher purity level. They also have a three month happiness guarantee, so 90 days, and if you aren't happy with the product they guarantee your money back. This product is considered organic.
- **Elixiol:** This brand has a great reputation or safety as well as high potency at an affordable price. This brand offers flavored or unflavored CBD oil and they have a potency range from mild to strong depending on the specific product. The price ranges from about forty dollars to over two hundred dollars depending on what you're looking for. Most people who use this brand take a thirty or thirty-five milligram dose twice daily.

Joint Pain & Rheumatoid Arthritis

For those of you who are lucky enough not to know, rheumatoid arthritis is a painful deformity that is caused by inflammation in the joints. It can cause pain in the fingers, feet, wrists, ankles and even causing swelling along inner body organs. Most people will develop this type of arthritis between twenty-five and forty-five, but it can affect children as young as three or four. Essentially pathogens wreck the tissue, causing inflammation to cause this disease. That inflammation attacks your joints and spreads to surrounding cartilage and bone. It can lead to immobility and can eventually cause a deformity in the joints, making it hard and painful to do every day activities. It can become crippling.

Various people will exhibit various symptoms, but they include pain, swelling, early morning stiffness in your joints, fatigue, muscular weakness and problems sleeping. You should see a doctor if you think you may have rheumatoid arthritis and see if you have the disease. It's best to start treatment early on. You're at a higher risk of this disease if you're female or your family as a history of rheumatoid arthritis. American Caucasians are also at a higher risk, and obesity can lead to a higher risk of the disease as well.

Normally cold, eat, and certain exercises are used to help decrease pain and stiffness, and you may need occupational therapy. Other methods are non-steroidal anti-inflammatory drugs, including ibuprofen. People who have more severe arthritis seek out pain management with a physician which leads them to damaging pain medication. Though, CBD oil has been proven to help with this disease because it alleviates inflammation of all types, including joint related inflammation. It also helps to manage chronic pain. Some CBD oils are better for this condition than others. Below you'll find some of the best CBD oils to treat rheumatoid arthritis.

- **Green Roads World:** This brand has a large array of CBD oils which are good for consumption or vaping depending on your preference. It is an affordable brand that ranges from about thirty to seventy dollars depending on the strength you're looking for, and it's considered to be a potent brand. Typically, people who use this brand will see pain reduction in as little as twenty minutes, and most people don't have to take more than thirty milligrams each day.

- **Pure Kana:** This is a top manufacturer of CBD oil, and it's extracted and it's considered to be more pure than other brands. It, of course, is a little more expensive. It ranges from around fifty dollars to one hundred and forty dollars depending on the potency you purchase. With this brand you usually don't need another brand, and it's also safe to take about thirty milligrams a day.

Chronic Pain

Everyone has pain, but that doesn't mean that you suffer from chronic pain. Chronic pain. Usually this is around the twelve week mark where they're constantly in pain, causing a change in your daily routine. Sadly, most treatments that are prescribed for chronic pain your body will eventually start to become accustomed to, and that will require you to continue to take a higher and higher dose. This can lead to various side effects, including risks to your gastrointestinal tract and other parts of the body. It can even become a costly treatment method that destroys your body instead of helping it to heal naturally. CBD oil is a potential answer to many.

To understand chronic pain, you need to understand what the most common causes of chronic pain are. Usually it's from an injury such as a muscle sprain which is due to a type of weakness, resulting in chronic pain which can affect your ability to eat and sleep. Sadly, little is known on how to eliminate chronic pain, especially since every case is different.

Recent studies have looked at how your brain actually processes pain to see if CBD oil can affect your brain. It's believed that CBD oil alters the way your body communicates pain so you can't "feel" it. When used orally, CBD oil has been shown to diminish neuropathic or even chronic inflammatory pain. You can also use CBD oil to help with pain that's related to cancer. Current treatments to cancer are generally considered toxic and it can weaken your body's cells.

Eye Health

CBD oil is not known to help with this nearly as much as cannabis oil, but cannabis oil can help with macular degeneration and glaucoma. Glaucoma, as you know, is an optic nerve disease that is actually caused by fluids building up in your eye. This means there is too much pressure on the lens, optic nerve and retina. It can lead to loss of vision or even blindness. Intraocular pressure is released with bot THC and CBD, but THC has shown to have a significant effect in reducing pressure which helps to prevent damage. Macular degeneration is a painless eye condition that's age related, and it's the loss of central vision. It makes it difficult to tell the difference between colors, recognize faces, and it makes it difficult to read. Once again, THC has been proven to help. Cannabis has proven to improve the connectivity between the postsynaptic neurons and photoreceptors, which helps you to receive light signals.

Improved Sleep

THC has been proven to help insomniacs, making cannabis oil a great choice for promoting healthier sleep schedules. THC, as we've discussed, has anti-anxiety properties which can help you to improve nighttime breathing problems as well as reduce sleep interruptions. Cannabis also helps to create a variety of focal sensory systems as well as direct neurotransmitter discharge, which will cause an expanded pleasure as well as a change in memory procedures. This can lead to improved sleep patterns as well. When people use cannabis oil for this purpose, they usually put two to three drops of cannabis oil in their drink before bed to start with.

Increased Heart Health

Cannabis oil can help keep your heart healthy by helping the cell reinforcement process which scrapes off the stores cholesterol from the heart. In turn it helps to strengthen your cardiovascular system overall, and it has antioxidant properties that help to protect your heart in the long term. The cannabinoids that are present in cannabis oil also relax and widen blood vessels which help to reduce blood pressure which in turns improves your circulation. This can help prevent heart conditions such as heart attack, hypertension and stroke. Two to three drops of cannabis oil in your drink three times a day is usually what people use to help protect their heart and improve heart related problems.

Better Appetite

If you have an eating disorder such as anorexia nervosa, cannabis oil can help. The THC and other cannabinoids normalize your body receptors to release hormones that help to tell you when you're hungry and increase your appetite. It'll help to improve your eating habits in the long term, and it's great if you're trying to regain some weight. THC ump starts mitochondria which makes your body demand nutrition, helping you to recover your urge to eat.

Helping with Weight Loss

What most people don't know is that if you're trying to lose weight, cannabis oil can help too because it has THCV. Even if you're increasing your calorie intake with cannabis oil, your body won't retain as much weight from it. For people hoping to get this result, it's best to stick with strains such as Doug's Varin, Master Kush or Cherry pie. If you're looking to use cannabis oil for weight loss it' good to take two to three drops before every meal. Usually its best about fifteen minutes before the meal, and it should have high levels of THC.

Stress Reduction

Any form of THC will help you with stress reduction. Stress is something everyone deals with, and it's a normal part of everyday life. However, if it's left unchecked it can cause serious health problems, which is where cannabis oil comes in handy. Cannabidiol oil helps to stimulate alpha waves, which occur naturally when someone is relaxed deeply. CBD Oil can also help to produce alpha waves, and CBD oil without having to experience that high. CBD oil can also help to calm overactive parts of your brain, helping to promote relaxation in another way.

Anxiety Relief

It's normal for everyone to feel anxious every once in a while. Some people however deal with chronic anxiety which can interfere with them completing day to day activities. Pharmaceutical medicines often have unwanted side effects, and yet they're treated like a one size fits all cure without working as effectively as they should. CBD is a side effect free, natural way to help reduce anxiety in most people. To start with it helps to reduce cortisol levels, and in another way it helps regulate serotonin. This will help with blood regulation.

Memory Enhancement

CBD is known to enhance memory if consumed on a regular basis. It can improve cognition as well. It helps to relax the mind so that you can make more connections, which means that it's beneficial for students, especially with a product that as a large amount of hemp oil too. Using CBD oil for this benefit is best in older people whose memory is already being affected by age, which is why it's so helpful with diseases such as Alzheimer's, but that isn't the only memory enhancing abilities it has.

Improved Motor Skills

Your motor skills are carried out after the brain and nervous systems tell your muscles to work in tandem. Therefore your motor skills can be enhanced through taking CBD oil on a regular basis. Motor skills begin to deteriorate overtime, which can lead to certain ailments, but CBD oil can be taken as a preventative measure.

Immune System Booster

CBD also helps with your immune system. Your immunity refers to your body's ability to fight disease. Through regular consumption of CBD supplements you can boost your body's natural immunity. CBD you can enhance your liver function which helps you to ward off different ailments. It also helps to keep your gut healthy which is also a great way to stave off common illnesses such as colds and coughs.

Fertility Help

CBD oil can also help to increase fertility, and many people find it to be an aphrodisiac which improves their libido. It's especially helpful to people who are having fertility issues. Just add a little CBD oil to your meals on a regular basis, and it can help to reverse infertility to a certain extent. You can also use CBD oil topically to the reproductive organs to help provide relief from fertility issues such as pain in those areas.

Healthy Bones

Many people neglect their bone health when they're trying to maintain their overall health, but bone health is vital. Bone health becomes even more important as you age. CBD supplements can help your body to absorb calcium into the bloodstream, which can keep your calcium from being depleted from your bones. If you have better bone health then you're less likely to suffer injuries that could shorten your lifespan or at least your quality of life.

Eczema

CBD oil can be used topically to help fight eczema, reducing the inflammation as well as the pain. So long as you use it topically, you'll be able to alleviate the pain within twenty to thirty minutes. You'll usually notice a large difference in two to three days, and for small cases it can clear up completely.

Varicose Veins

CBD oil can be used to help treat varicose veins as well. Varicose veins can often be found on the legs, and it's due to circulatory problems. If you've ever suffered from this, then you know that it's painful. CBD oil can be used to relieve the swelling, pain, heaviness, and visibility of your varicose veins when made into a topical cream.

CBD Oil Products

Here is a look at some CBD oil products that you might want to use.

CBD Oil Creams

When you're using CBD oil in a cream, you're using a lotion that's been infused with oil. This is applied to the area you're trying to target. You'll want to use it for soreness, inflammation or pain. It's great for sports related injuries, but it can also help with headaches, dermatitis, and even itching. CBD cream doesn't penetrate into your bloodstream. Instead, it reacts with the CB2 receptors in your body. You'll find that some CBD oils are prepared with cayenne or mint to help with certain symptoms.

CBD Oil Capsules

Many people believe that CBD oil capsules is easier, and many people assume it's safer because it's in pre-measured doses. If you struggle with dosing, then this is a great alternative. Its convenience is the best part of CBD oil capsules, and it's great for stress relief, anxiety or pain management as well as any other condition you'd take CBD oil in an ingestible form for. It's a fast delivery method, and it's a great choice if you don't like the taste of CBD oil.

CBD Oil Tinctures

Tinctures are a common CBD product, and it's a liquid that you put under your tongue or mix into your drink or food. This is an affordable option, and it's a great way to try the product for the first time. It offers a low concentration of CBD, and it's commonly used for insomnia, depression and anxiety.

CBD Oil Candy & Gum

Candy or gum can also be used, and one brand of CBD oil gum is CanChew. It helps to treat various symptoms including nausea, vomiting, anxiety and pain. It's a highly effective way to use CBD since it comes into direct contact with the mucosal membranes, which allows your body to absorb it quickly.

Vaping CBD Oil

This is a delivery method that is growing in popularity. CBD enters the lungs and diffuses into your bloodstream directly before passing through your liver and gut. The first-pass effect is mostly from it traveling through your gut wall and the liver, and there is a fraction of the drug that's lost before reaching your systemic circulation. However, when you vape CBD oil, this isn't a worry. This means that the CBD gets into your system faster, which is great for nausea and anxiety which you'll want to get rid of quickly. You'll also use less CBD at one time when you can use the effects immediately.

CBD Oil Patches

This is another topical method of CBD, but it does allow it to penetrate into the bloodstream. The patch is a medicated adhesive which is placed over your skin to give you a specific dose through your skin and into your bloodstream. It promotes healing to an injured area, and it provides a controlled release of CBD. It's done through a porous membrane or through body heat which melts the medication which is embedded in the adhesive, which your body then absorbs. It's best to use this method when using CBD to treat inflammation or pain.

CBD Oil Spray

The first thing you need to know about CBD oil as a spray is that it has an incredibly low concentration. This is why it's one of the least recommended ways to take CBD oil. Usually each spray will carry between one to three milligrams of CBD oil, and it's difficult to measure how much you're taking. The measurements can be off, and it won't help with most pain related ailments.

CBD Oil & General Dosage

If you've decided that you want to take CBD oil, you're probably wondering how much you should take each day. CBD oil specialists say it depends on your tolerance, body size and the level of pain you're experiencing. This means that there isn't direct scientific information that will tell you the exact amount you should be taking. It's a natural remedy, so you should slowly up your dose as needed.

However, the FDA says that you should handle it as you do food, so it will come with serving size information. However, this probably isn't right for what you're using it for. So you'll need to experiment with the dosage to see how little you need to take to help alleviate your pain or symptoms. Different brands will also state that you should take a certain amount as well as how many milligrams that dose contains.

So, if one brand requires ten drops as a serving size, this is usually only five milligrams of CBD oil. However, you may discover that through trial and error you need double this per day to alleviate your own symptoms, and you'd adjust the serving accordingly. Of course, take your weight into consideration as well. If you're heavier, you'll often need more than if you're skinnier.

Minor Pain

If your baby is experiencing minor pain, and is under 25 pounds, you shouldn't give them any more than 4.5 mg. if the child weighs between 26 and 45 pounds, then you can start around 6 mg. if the weight of the child is between 86 and 150, then you can use 12 mg. between the weight of 151 and 240, 18 mg is usually best. If you're over 240 lbs., then 22.5 mg is best for minor pain.

Moderate Pain

For 25 pounds, you'll want to take 6 mg. between 25 and 45 pounds, you'd want to opt for 9 mg. for someone weighting between 46 and 84 pounds, 12 mg is recommended. If you're between 86 and 150 pounds, then try 15 mg. if you weight between 151 to 240 pounds, 22.5 mg is best, and when you're over 240 pounds, taking 30 mg is recommended.

Severe Pain

For someone below 25 pounds experiencing severe pain, it's recommended that you take 9 mg. for someone between 26 and 45 pounds, 12 mg is recommended for this type of pain. If you're between 46 to 85, then try 15 mg. if you're between 86 and 150, try 19 mg. if you're between 151 and 240, 27 mg is recommended. For anyone over 24 pounds, 45 mg is recommended for severe pain.

CBD Oil Extraction Methods

If you're going to be making your own CBD oil at home or you just want to know more about the way CBD oil is made to better understand the product, this chapter is going to help. We'll cover the best extraction methods as well as the most common ones used in this chapter. The goal of extract is considered simple. All you want to do is pull the cannabinoid out and make sure it comes in a highly concentrated form that's also suitable to be consumed. Just make sure that you have a plant that's rich in CBD, which is covered later in this book. Even if you're just buying CBD oil, you'll learn which strains are the best base.

CO2 Cannabis Extraction

This is an extraction method that can be divided into three different categories. You have supercritical, subcritical and mid-critical. Supercritical is what's most commonly used when it comes to the CO2 method. It uses pressurized carbon dioxide to pull the CBD away from the cannabis plant. It acts as a solvent, and it's considered both effective and safe. The equipment you use is effective as well.

This isn't a method you'll want to use at home, but you can look up to see if the method has been used in the CBD oil you're buying. It requires machines that are able to freeze CO2 gas and then compress it until it turns into a cold liquid state. That liquid is then taken and the temperature is increased as well as the pressure until it becomes supercritical which means that it's capable of adopting properties between a gas and liquid simultaneously. CO2 in its supercritical state is great for chemical extract because it doesn't cause damage or denaturing that would make the product unfit to be consumed.

The liquid CO2 is raised to a higher pressure due to a compressor, but other people use a heater. The next step involves your high-quality cannabis, and then the CO2 pulls the essential oils from the plant. This method is incredibly expensive, and most of the equipment will cost $40,000. It's a complex method that should be left to the professionals.

Olive Oil Method

This is considered to be a beginner friendly method of CBD extraction. This is great if you want to do your own CBD oil extraction. The first thing you need to do is make sure that you have raw cannabis, making sure that you have a strain high in CBD. Just remember that strains that are high in CBD does not necessarily mean that they are low in THC so research your strain carefully. You have to heat your plant material to a specific temperature for a specific length of time, and this activates the plant's natural chemicals. You want to heat the plant to 284 degrees for thirty minutes.

After that, you add in your olive oil, heating it to 212 degrees for two hours. This will result in the extraction of the CBD oil you want. It's a safe method that also isn't very expensive. You can usually use what's in your kitchen! The biggest problem is that you need to realize the resulting CBD infused oil is perishable, so once you're done making it you need to store it properly in a cool, dark place. Make sure that it's stored in an airtight container. It also will only yield a small amount of CBD infused oil, so it's the wrong choice for any company. This extraction method is for personal use only.

Solvent Extraction

This is great for smaller scale oil product, and it doesn't cost too much either. You can easily obtain the equipment, and it's a simple process to follow. The solvents are usually butane, grain alcohol, isopropyl alcohol, ethanol and hexane. Some people do consider this to be a dangerous process due to the flammable substances that are used. The least recommended solvents on that list are butane and pure grain alcohol. Using a highly flammable solvent can destroy the therapeutic plant waxes that make CBD oil medicinal.

You'll need one drip coffee maker, a few paper coffee filters, a lighter, a glass bowl, a plastic spoon, a fine strainer, a large bowl, sixteen ounces of isopropyl alcohol, a home water distiller machine, and an ounce of dried cannabis. Start by mixing your alcohol with your dried cannabis in your glass bowl. Mix it using a plastic spoon, allowing it to soak for a few minutes. You can then use the strainer to separate the solid from the liquids. Place a paper coffee filter inside your coffee maker, but don't turn on your coffee maker yet.

Pour the liquid through, letting it drip, and this will spate the fine dust of cannabis from your liquid. Once you have your liquid, you can use the water distiller to separate the ethanol from your oil. Once the oil has been separated, you can pour it into a glass bowl, placing it in the coffee pot warmer. Turn the coffee maker on now, allowing the glass bowl to heat up. Give it time to let the ethanol particles evaporate.

Let it sit for a few hours, and the end product should be a dark brown color that's thick and oily. This substances should be pure CBD oil when done properly. Make sure that there is no ethanol left in there! You should be able to dip a paperclip into the liquid and then try to light it with a lighter. If it catches fire, then you have to leave it on the coffee pot for a few more hours.

Some CBD Oil Health Recipes

You can usually purchase topical creams that already come with CBD oil in them, but sometimes it's better and cheaper to make the product yourself with the CBD oil you already have. This way you know exactly what's going into the product that you're using. It allows you to personalize the smell, make the right amount you need, and even cut down on packaging and plastic.

CBD Salve

Ingredients:

- 1/3 Cup Jojoba Oil
- 1 1/3 Cup Coconut Oil
- 10 Drops Lavender Essential Oil
- 1/3 Cup Beeswax, Grated
- 3 Tablespoon Cocoa Butter
- 1 Cup Aloe Vera
- 9 Grams Dried Cannabis, Ground

Directions:

1. Start by preheating your oven to 240. Spread your dried cannabis on a baking sheet after it's been ground. Once your oven is preheated, allow it to decarboxylase in the oven for a half hour.
2. While your cannabis is in the oven, get out a saucepan and add in your jojoba oil and your coconut oil, and ten heat it over low heat while stirring constantly. It should melt and mix together.
3. Once you're done baking your cannabis, take it out of the oven, adding it into the oil mixture. Allow your oil to continue to cook on low heat, and then stir constantly for twenty-five minutes. If you don't contagiously stir you're risking burning your cannabis which will ruin your batch.
4. Remove the mix from heat, and then use a cheesecloth to strain it.
5. Add your beeswax, heating it until it's melted. As it melts, you'll want to stir your coconut oil back into the mixture, and then mix in your essential oils too. After everything is mixed together remove it from heat.

6. Immediately add in your aloe Vera gel and cocoa butter, stirring well.
7. Store in a jar, and use as needed.

Stiffness Oil

Ingredients:

- 50 mg CBD Oil
- 10 Drops Eucalyptus Essential Oil
- 2 Tablespoons Olive Oil

Directions:

1. Start by mixing all ingredients together, and then store it in a squeeze bottle.
2. Massage over any stiff area.

Neck Pain & Arthritis Lotion

Ingredients:

- 1 ½ Teaspoons Beeswax, Grated
- 12 Drops Lavender Essential Oil
- 20 mg CBD Oil
- 2 Teaspoon Shea Butter

Directions:

1. Start by putting your beeswax and shea butter in a bowl before microwaving it for a minute. Add in your CBD Oil and then add in your essential oils, stirring well.
2. Pour this mixture into a container, allowing it to set. Allow it to harden before using it.

Eczema Balm

Ingredients:

- 1 ½ Teaspoons CBD Oil
- 10 Drops Lavender Essential Oil
- 1 ½ Teaspoons Shea Butter
- 1 ½ Teaspoons Beeswax, Grated

Directions:

1. Start by melting your shea butter and beeswax in a microwave safe bowl for a full minute.
2. Stir in your lavender essential oil and CBD oil.
3. Pour it into a desired container, and set it to the side to cool. Once hardened, use it topically as desired.

Varicose Vein Oil

Ingredients:

- 1 ½ Ounces CBD Oil
- 20-25 Drops Cypress Essential Oils
- 20-25 Drops Immortelle Essential Oil

Directions:

1. Mix together, and apply to the area, rubbing it in gently twice daily.

Body Butter

Ingredients:

- 1/3 Cup Coconut Oil
- 1/3 Cup Magnesium Oil
- 15 Drops Peppermint Essential Oil
- ½ Cup Cocoa Butter
- 40 mg CBD Oil

Directions:

1. Start by adding your coconut oil and cocoa butter to a saucepan before placing it over medium heat. Melt it together, stirring so

that it mixes well. Once completely melted and mixed, then remove the mixture from heat.

2. Add in your peppermint essential oil and magnesium, and then add in your CBD oil. Stir well, letting the mixture cool.
3. Once cool, whip the mixture with a hand mixer until light and fluffy. Use this for aches and pains.

CBD Oil Food Recipes

Remember that CBD oil can be taken for heart health, healthy bones, better immune function, better brain function, and other medical benefits that require it to be taken as a preventive method. You can do this with tasty CBD oil infused food recipes!

CBD Brownies

Ingredients:

- 1 Cup Oil
- 1 Gram CBD Isolate, 99%
- 1 Cup White Sugar
- 1/3 Cup Cocoa Powder
- ¼ Teaspoon Baking Powder
- 1 Teaspoon Vanilla Extract, Pure
- 2 Eggs
- ½ Cup Flour

Directions:

1. Start by heating your oven to 350, and then mix your CBD Isolate with oil, mixing it in with your sugar. Make sure it's blended well.
2. Add in your vanilla and eggs, stirring it until it's mixed thoroughly.
3. Mix all of your dry ingredients in a different bowl, making sure it's mixed all the way.
4. Stir in your dry ingredients into your liquid mixture, and pour it into a greased nine by nine pan.
5. Allow it to bake for twenty minutes. Your brownies will contain 24.75 mg of CBD when cut into nine pieces.

Peanut Brittle

Ingredients:

- ¼ Teaspoon Sea Salt, Fine

- ½ Cup Light Corn Syrup
- ¼ Cup Water
- 1 Cup White Sugar
- 4 ½ Tablespoons Oil
- 1 Teaspoon Baking Soda
- 1 Cup Peanuts, Chopped
- ¼ Gram CBD Isolate

Directions:

1. Use a double boiler, brining your oil to a boil and add in your sugar while stirring frequently. Remove it from heat once all of your sugar is dissolved.
2. Add your infused isolate, and then add in a teaspoon of baking soda, mixing well. Pour this onto a greased baking pan. Some people add optional berries or chocolate chips at this stage. Allow the mixture to cool, and then after an hour, break and serve.

Matcha Latte

Ingredients:

- 1 Cup Hot Water
- 1 Teaspoon Matcha Powder
- 2 Teaspoons Honey
- 1 Teaspoon CBD Oil
- ¼ Cup Coconut Milk, Full Fat

Directions:

1. Blend everything together until smooth, and then place it in a mug. Enjoy warm.

Soft Peanut Butter Cookies

Ingredients:

- 2 Eggs, Large
- 1 ½ Cups Creamy Peanut Butter

- 1 Cup Coconut Oil, Softened
- 1 Gram CBD Isolate, 99%
- 2 Cups Flour
- 2 Tablespoons Vanilla Extract, Pure
- 2 Teaspoons Baking Soda
- 4 Teaspoon Cornstarch
- ½ Teaspoon Sea Salt, Fine

Directions:

1. Strat by combining your isolate with your coconut oil. Use a stand mixture to combine your coconut oil mixture, eggs, sugar and peanut butter.
2. Use medium-high to cream the mixture until it's fluffy and whipped. Make sure that the sides of the bowl have been scraped down and incorporated into it.
3. Add in your vanilla, beating for another minute.
4. Add your cornstarch, baking soda, flour and sea salt. Mix again for a full minute.
5. Use a cookie scoop, forming mounds and placing them on a large plate. Cover the tray, wrapping it in plastic, and then allow it to sit in the fridge for two hours.
6. Let your dough sit out for fifteen to twenty minutes before you cook.
7. Heat your oven to 350, and then put the dough on a lined baking sheet. Make sure that you have two inches between each one.
8. Allow your cookies to bake for seven to nine minutes. The tops should be set.
9. Allow your cookies to cook for ten minutes on the baking sheet, and then you can store them for up to a week in an airtight container. You can freeze them for up to three minutes. You can also freeze the dough for up to three months before it's cooked.

Chocolate Macaroons

Ingredients:

- 3 Tablespoons Coconut Crème, Melted

- 3 Tablespoons Cacao Butter
- 3 Tablespoons Water, Warm
- 3 Tablespoons Hemp Butter
- 1 ½ Cup Coconut, Shredded
- 5 Tablespoons Cacao Powder
- 7-8 Drops Stevia
- 3 Tablespoons Xylitol
- 2 Pinches Sea Salt, Fine

Directions:

1. Get out a double boiler, and then place your water in a bowl, whisking in your coconut crème, hemp butter, cacao butter, water, stevia, salt, and xylitol.
2. Sift your cacao powder, adding it into your mixture. Stir well, and then add in your shredded coconut.
3. Stir all ingredients together until it's combined well.
4. Use a miniature ice cream scoop, putting them on a baking sheet lined with parchment paper.
5. Allow it to chill in the fridge for hour hours, allowing it to firm. You can store this in the fridge for up to a week.

Chocolate Chip Cookies

Ingredients:

- 2/3 Cup Cannabis Coconut Oil, Liquid
- 1 ¼ Cup Coconut Sugar
- 2 Tablespoons Spring Water
- ½ Cup Almond Milk, Unsweetened
- 1 Tablespoon Arrowroot Starch
- 2 Cups All Purpose Flour
- 1 Teaspoon Vanilla Extract, Pure
- 2/3 Cup Cocoa Powder, Raw
- 1 Cup Chocolate Chips
- 1 Teaspoon Baking Soda
- ½ Teaspoon Sea Salt, Fine
- ¼ Cup Brown Sugar

Directions:

1. Start by heating your oven to 375, and then grease a baking sheet.
2. Mix your cannabis coconut oil, almond milk, sugar, brown sugar, water, arrowroot starch, water, and vanilla in a bowl. Set it to the side.
3. Mix in your chocolate chips, flour, cocoa powder, sea salt and baking soda in a different bowl, making sure it's well combined.
4. Add your flour mixture into your oil mixture slowly, making sure it's well blended.
5. Start by forming your dough into one inch balls, placing them about two inches apart before placing them on your baking sheet.
6. Bake them in your oven for ten minutes, and ten allow them to sit on your baking sheet for five minutes.
7. Transfer your cookies to a wire rack, allowing them to cool before serving them.

Strawberry Smoothie

Ingredients:

- 3 Tablespoons Coconut Oil
- 2 Tablespoon Hemp Seed
- 2 Tablespoons Chia Gel
- 1 Tablespoon Hemp Oil
- 6 Strawberries, Frozen
- 1 Tablespoon Honey, Raw
- 2 Cups Almond Milk, Original

Directions:

1. Throw all ingredients into a blender, and then blend for three minutes before serving.

Carrot Cake

Ingredients:

Cake:

- 2 Cups All Purpose Flour
- 2 Teaspoons Cinnamon
- 1 Teaspoon Baking Soda
- ¼ Teaspoon Sea Salt, Fine
- 3 Eggs
- 1 Cup Hemp Oil
- ¾ Cup Buttermilk
- 1 ½ Cups Sugar
- 2 ½ Cups Carrots, Shredded
- 2 Teaspoons Vanilla Extract, Pure
- 1 Cup Flaked Coconut
- 1 Cup Walnuts, Chopped
- 1 Cup Raisins

Frosting:

- ½ Cup Butter, Softened (or CBD Butter)
- 1 Cup Cream Cheese
- 4 Cups Powdered Sugar
- 1 Teaspoon Vanilla Extract, Pure

Directions:

1. Start by preheating your oven to 350 degrees.
2. Sift your baking soda, sea salt, cinnamon, and flour together before placing it in a medium bowl. Set it to the side.
3. Combine your buttermilk, your oil mixture, eggs, vanilla and sugar in a different bowl, mixing again.
4. Add your oil mixture into your flour mixture, making sure it's well combined.
5. Combine your coconut, shredded carrots, walnuts and raisins in a different bowl.
6. Add your carrot mix into the batter mix, making sure it's mixed thoroughly.
7. Place your batter in a greased pan, allowing it to bake for an hour. A toothpick should be able to be inserted into it and come out clean. Remove your cake, and then allow it to cool.
8. While your cake cooks, take your cream cheese, butter, sugar and

vanilla, beating it until creamy and smooth to make your frosting.
9. Frost your cake once it's cooled, and stir it in the fridge.

Cannabis Strains

If you're looking for cannabis oil, you should be getting it from a strain that can produce high quality oil. With cannabis oil, you're looking for THC, so you should get it from a strain that produces high levels of THC, which is where this chapter comes in handy.

Sour Diesel Strain

This is also known as the NY Diesel strain because it originally comes from New York City, and it is a sativa dominant hybrid, so it has 16-20% THC levels. However, it has low levels of CBD. It has a sweet lime smell and taste, and to some degree it can cause paranoia. However, it also helps to energize you, helping to make you more social and outgoing with a small body high that often lasts for two to three hours. It can help with stress, anxiety, chronic pain, nausea, and depression.

Vanilla Kush

This is an Indica dominant strain with 20% levels of THC. It has a low level of CBD about 1.2%. It has a vanilla smell that's smooth and sweet and a vanilla taste that gets stronger when you vape it. This produces an oil that will leave you uplifted, happy, relaxed, euphoric and sleepy. It's ideal for treating pain, insomnia, lack of appetite, depression and stress.

White Rhino

This is an indica dominant strain that has 14-20% THC levels with 1% CBD and 1% CBN levels. It has an earthy and bitter smell, and it's considered to have a spicy woody taste. It produces euphoria, happiness, relaxation, and a sleepy feeling. This is why it's great for treating stress, chronic pain, insomnia, depression and bipolar disorder.

Orange Hill

This is from a blend of the orange bud as well as the California orange, and it a half and half strain. That means its 50% sativa and 50% indica. It has a high level of THC at 21%, and it has a 2% CBD level. It's considered to have an off orange taste and smell. This is a strain that's great for giving you euphoria, helping you be social, and it can make you feel "giggly drunk". It can also make some people feel hungry and sleepy. It's best for treating depression, stress and insomnia.

Amnesia Haze (Feminized)

This is a sativa dominant strain with high levels of THC at 20-25%. It has less than 10% CBD, and it has an earthy flavor with hints of citrus. It provides a high feeling that usually kicks in after about fifteen minutes, but this effect doesn't last long. It can help with depression, ease nausea, ease fears, and help with migraines.

More Cannabis Strains & High CBD

We've briefly talked about cannabis strains in this book, but in this chapter we'll take a more in depth look so that you can find what you need without too much trouble. All of these strains have high levels of CBD, so they'll help you medically more than just normal strains of cannabis which produce a high. However, you need to understand that these are cannabis strains that have high CBD, so they will have THC as well. Only buy these strains if they are legal in your area.

Harlequin

This strain has high CBD, and t has an earthy smell that has a hint of oak. It's sativa dominant, so it'll help increase your alertness while easing anxiety. It's also great for pain management or those suffering from migraines. The CBD to THC ration is 5:2.

Sweet & Sour Widow

This is a White Widow strain that's been enriched with CBD, and it has a 1:1 ratio of THC and CBD. It's considered to be sweet and woodsy, and it's read for pain reduction. It also works great for relieving fatigue and promoting sleep. Other people take it for depression.

Ringo's Gift

This is a hybrid of AC-DC and Harle-Tsu strains, so it's almost completely THC free! The ratio is actually 24:1 with CBD being the highest. It's considered citrus and piney, and it relieves pain quickly. It's great for reducing inflammation, helping with muscle pain and help with headaches.

Pennywise

This is a strain that's been breed for insomnia as well as chronic pain. It was made from Harlequin and Jack the Ripper. It has a CBD to THC ratio of 1:1, and it has a peppery smell.

Harle-Tsu

This is a hybrid of Sour Tsunami and Harlequin, and the CBD to THC ration is 20:1, so it has almost no THC in it. It's also considered woodsy and citrusy, and it helps people suffering from chronic depression. You will not experience a strong high if you experience any at all. It helps to relax you, so most people take it before bed.

AC/DC

This is a sativa dominant strain, and helps to treat severe multiple sclerosis. That is the best use of this strain, and it should be used to treat severe cases.

Catonic

This is a hybrid mixture of G13 Haze and MK Ultra. This strain has significant effects on the body to promote relaxation. That's why this is a great strain or people who are suffering from chronic anxiety. It helps to uplift your mood, so don't let the name scare you away. The feelings that this strain produces help to naturally reduce stress and fight fatigue as well by giving you the energy boost you need.

Sour Tsunami

This strain was one of the first that was grown to specifically cultivate CBD over THC. If you suffer from a high amount of depression or stress, then this can be a great strain for you. It gives most people a more positive outlook by promoting more relaxation. It has a sweet smell, so more people tend to like it than other strains available.

Cannabis Effects

Like everything, there are some side effects that you need to look out for when ingesting any cannabis product, including CBD products. THC usually comes with a euphoric high, which is why many people like to smoke marijuana. It can also produce relaxation and reduce your stress overall. It can also cause some people to hallucinate. It can also reduce pain, ease social anxiety, and it can increase introspection and creativity depending on the person.

CBD usually prevents hallucinations when taken with THC. It can also reduce the paranoia that THC produces. CBD can help to ease anxiety and relieve pain when used alone as well. Just remember that each strain of cannabis will have different results because some are more intense than others. Each strain is derived from two types of cannabis plants indica or sativa. Stavia strains are considered to be more "fun" strains, and they're usually paired for social engagements or during something that you want to be creative with. However, indica strains are meant to help you to relax, and it's used for depression and anxiety. Indica strains can also help with insomnia, PTSD and more.

Recreational and medical effects of CBD

Here are a few recreational and medical effects of CBD that are positive.

- Slower progression of disease or cancer
- Anxiety relief
- Nausea relief
- Pain relief
- Euphoria
- Increased creativity
- Increased agreeableness
- Increased introspection
- Increased sensation
- Increased sociability
- Increased libido
- A feeling of well-being
- Altered perceptions

- Overall feeling of calm

Side effects of CBD

- Irritated or red eyes
- Panic attacks
- Increased thirst
- Ataxia or lethargy
- Increased appetite
- Increased heart rate
- Dry eye
- Forgetfulness
- Dry eye
- Depersonalization
- Dizziness
- Coughing
- Bronchitis
- Anxiety or paranoia

Just remember while not everyone will experience all medicinal benefits they also won't experience all of the side effects. For most people, the side effects are limited to what you see joked about on TV, such as the munchies or red eyes. Eye drops and healthy snacks can help you to get past them. Cannabis also isn't lethal unless you're allergic to it. It's considered to be the safest medicinal product currently on the market, and it's virtually impossible to overdose on it.

It is extremely rare for people to truly become addicted to cannabis or marijuana as well. What people develop occasionally is called dependency, especially if they're using it to treat a condition such as insomnia. This dependency isn't considered as unhealthy as a dependency on sleeping pills or alcohol would be.

Cannabis doesn't have any negative effects on your kidney or liver, so it doesn't have long-term health concerns other than chronic bronchitis. This can be avoided by not smoking cannabis. This is why it's considered to be one of the safest treatment options on the market on the time, no matter if you're using THC or CBD.

Getting a Medical Marijuana Card

If you are in a state where medicinal marijuana is legal, then you may want to try to get a medical marijuana card. There are slightly different regulations regarding a marijuana card depending on the state that you're in, and they all have different conditions that will qualify you for one. The first thing you need is a diagnosis from a medical professional for a qualifying condition. Just remember that your doctor cannot give you a marijuana card, and they can't prescribe the card to you. Your doctor can only document your condition and provide you with that diagnosis and documentation. They can also give you a medical marijuana card application.

Illnesses & Conditions

Most states have the following illnesses and conditions in common as far as qualifying you for a medical marijuana card.

- Epilepsy or Seizures
- Muscle Spasm Disorders
- HIV
- Hepatitis C
- Multiple Sclerosis
- Glaucoma
- Crohn's Disease
- Chronic Pain
- Cancer
- Chronic Nausea
- Cachexia
- Alzheimer's Disease
- AIDS
- ALS

You'll want to contact your state's Department of Health and do research online to make sure you know your state's specific qualifying conditions for Medical Marijuana use.

Step 1: See a Doctor

You'll want an established physical patient relationship so that you can document your condition. This doctor can be a traditional doctor (MD), an osteopathic doctor (DO), a homeopathic doctor (MD/H or OD/H) or a naturopathic doctor (NMD or ND).

Step 2: Get Your Form Signed

Once you've established a relationship with a physical, you'll need them to complete and sign a Medical Marijuana Certification form. You can't use some random form online, so make sure you get the one that's specific to your state. Also, keep in mind a written recommendation won't be enough. It has to be the official state-certified form. Keep in mind that just because the physician you're currently seeing didn't diagnose you with your condition, they can still sign the form for you. They just need to have access to your previous medical records to verify that you have the condition for it to be legal.

Step 3: Collect Your Documentation

After you've had your state certification form signed, you can collect your documentation to complete the rest of your paperwork. You'll have to get proof of residency in your state. You can use a driver's license, passport, or any other state or even federally issued photo identification that you have. You often need to provide a current photograph of yourself within the last sixty days of your application as well.

In the photo you take you can't have hats, glasses or anything else that could obscure the view of your face. You can get this officially taken at any place that does passport photos, since they have the same regulations. If you get SNAP (Supplemental Nutrition Assistance Program, also commonly called Food stamps), you will have to provide documentation of your current eligibility and benefits.

Step 4: Turn Them into PDFs

You'll need to scan all of the documents into a PDF format, which will allow you to upload tem into your state's website. You can then submit them with your Patient Attestation Form.

Step 5: Register with the Department of Health

You'll have to then register with your states specific Department of Health, and make sure that you submit all of your documents and certified forms. For most states, you can do this online. Though, some states do require that you do this by mail.

How Much it Costs

Getting a medical marijuana a card isn't free, but the exact price will depend on the state you're in. on average, an application fee is about $150, but if you receive SNAP benefits, then you can usually get this fee reduced. When it's reduced, it can be about $75-$100. This isn't the only fee though. There is usually an additional fee for the registry identification card, which costs about $200. This means you'll likely pay $350 total, and you can pay another $100-$200 in doctor's fee.

So, you'll want to budget around $500-$750 to obtain your card. You'll also need to prepare for the cost of your medical marijuana, as many products can be expensive. You'll want to check local dispensaries to get the right prices for your area. You may also want to travel to a larger city that has multiple dispensaries to ensure the best competitive price. These fees do not include the normal fees that doctors' visits will cost to become established with your doctor, getting your photo, or even obtaining a new license or other documentation.

Opening a Dispensary?

If you want to open a dispensary, you'll need to budget a lot more. The fees are high. You'll spend about $500 to register as a dispensary agent, and it costs about $5,000 for the registration certificate. It can then cost $1,000 to renew the certificate, and $2,500 if you have to move to a different location. This is just an example of a few of the fees involved.

What to Keep In Mind

The key points that you should take away from this is as follows

- **It Isn't Easy:** It's not as easy as just telling your doctor you have anxiety and them writing you a marijuana prescription.

- **You Can't Purchase in a Different State:** If you are in a state that doesn't allow for medical marijuana, you cannot purchase marijuana in another state and bring it back home with you. This will count as drug trafficking, which is a federal crime.
- **Don't Purchase Recreational Marijuana:** If you already have a medical marijuana card, you can't go to a different state and purchase recreational marijuana and bring it home with you. This would also be considered drug trafficking.
- **It's Only Valid for Your State:** A medical marijuana card is only valid for the state that it was issued to you in.
- **Don't Cross State Lines:** Even with a medical marijuana card, you shouldn't cross state lines with legally purchased marijuana. It is a risk, as it will come into question if it's being transported for a particular use, which could lead to you being charged with a crime.

Buying CBD Oil

You know that if you want to buy cannabis oil, you'll need a medical marijuana card. So, let's now concentrate on how to practically find the right CBD oil for you. It may seem easy, and you may think that you can just go online and find whatever promises the best result, but there are many scams and dangers out there.

Deciding Quality

There are thousands of places and companies that provide CBD out there, and less than half of them will actually give you a good, high quality product. It's important to be discriminating. While high quality is important in most products, it's crucial when it comes to picking out CBD. Low quality CBD may contain dangerous substances and impurities. You may even end up buying high THC products which might be illegal where you are, but either way you'd be held responsible. You should stick to vendors that are certified, such as Healthy Hemp Oil or some of the other brands that have been named in this book so far. Stick with companies that invest in third-party lab tests are US manufacturers. If you're informed, then you can walk away a happy customer.

The Price

When you are looking for a car and find an amazing car that sounds perfect at an oddly cheap price, then you know that there's likely something seriously wrong with it. This is usually the case with CBD too. CBD oil is an expensive product, so stay away from anything that seems suspiciously cheap. It may contain stuff in it that you don't want to ingest. Making CBD oil isn't a cheap process, so if you're buying something cheap, you're likely getting scammed out of your money. When looking at the price, you need to think about it as an investment. With the right price, you will be getting what you both want and deserve in the product.

Some Buying Criteria

When you start looking at CBD products you'll see they come in various sizes, forms and shapes. There are three major things you need to look for when you are looking at a product to see if it's right for you.

- **Volume:** You need to see how much CBD is in a product before you buy it. Different products will contain different quantities of CBD. You aren't going to find a product that has "too much CBD" in it. It just is important that you know how much CBD you're ingesting so you can find out what does and doesn't work for you without taking more than you need.
- **Hemp Oil Volume:** When you're looking at CBD products, you are going to be looking at two different types of quantities. You're going to look to see how much CBD is contained in the product, and you'll want to see how much hemp oil is contained in the product. Remember that hemp oil is healthy for you but it doesn't have the same medicinal benefits of CBD oil. Think about it like you would a fish oil supplement. Fish oil supplements have fish oil and then a beneficial compound called DHA and EPA. You'll want to know the total for EPA and DHA per each capsule. You aren't looking for total fish oil. It's the same way with CBD products. How much hemp oil and how much CBD oil is in the product since both are beneficial to each other.
- **Concentration:** Concentration is just as important as the volume of CBD oil. Concentration is in regards to the abundance of CBD once it's compared to the volume of the product as a whole. You'll find products that range from normal strength to high CBD concentrations. What concentration you end up choosing will depend on what product you're taking and what you're trying to cheat. If you're just starting, remember the recommended doses and then only scale up if you need to.

Tailoring it to You

You need to ask yourself what type of CBD product is going to work best for what you need. Some CBD products come in different flavors and formats, so you need to ask yourself if you're looking for a fast and easy solution. You should also ask yourself if you want it to be as flavorful and fun as possible. If you aren't looking for special flavors or fun, then it becomes easier to find a CBD oil that's right for you, but it's less easy if you're actively trying to avoid flavors altogether. CBD oil has a natural flavor that many people do not like.

Conclusion

Now you know everything you need to get started with CBD or cannabis oil to meet your medicinal needs. It doesn't matter if you're using it for preventative use or for a specific condition, with this CBD and cannabis oil guide, you should know enough to find the right option for you. Just keep in mind that each strain is different, so it's important that you know where your CBD oil or cannabis oil comes from before you use it. Do your research, and remember that if the price is too cheap, then it's likely too good to be true.